Health Care Information Technology
The Hardware and Software Focus:
Critical Factors for Medical Systems Implementation
2nd Edition

ISBN 978-0-615-44776-6

Printed in the United States of America

First Printing, 2011

Second Edition 2011

For permission requests and ordering information: Write to the publisher,
addressed "Attention: Book Coordinator," at the address below.

HCITSC LLC
P.O. Box 3388
Federal Way, WA 98063

How to Use this Book

Attention Health Care, Health Information Management, and Health Care Information Technology Industry: Regardless of what stage you are in with your organization's EMR, revenue cycle, payment processing, and/or medical systems implementation, you can benefit from this book. What you are about to read is an attempt to demystify common sources of confusion and to shed light on solutions to typical problems. Many in the industry are purchasing this book to help provide an understanding of the following critical factors of Medical Systems Implementations:

- Business planning of Medical Systems Implementation
- Essential misunderstandings related to terminology
- How to access funds allocated through ARRA (the American Recovery and Reinvestment Act)
- How to hire for key positions
- Implementation costs (with clear examples)
- Industry definitions through our handy guide
- Key legislation that affects the industry
- Potential pathways to entering the Health Care Information Technology field
- Specific IT hardware and software required, as well as security requirements

... and much, much more!

This book can also be used as an educational reference to get up to speed before taking on a new position or before taking a course on health care-related topics. No matter what your current job may be, this book can help you move forward in the health care field.

And look for more books on related health care topics from HC-IT-SC in the near future!

Reasons for 2nd Edition 2011

The author and HC-IT-SC want to begin by apologizing to those who purchased the first edition. Considering that author and HC-IT-SC intentions is to provide the field with assistance in a constructive way, please do not hesitate to write the author with your concerns if you see that any of our books have been incorrectly presented. We will fix it immediately and send you a corrected copy. This revised edition corrects and improves upon the original volume by offering a more positive message to those in the health care industry. This book is intended to serve as a reference guide for all, presenting a constructive perspective on the health care industry and its many components. Creating and adding to this book should be a community effort. Please feel free to provide data to improve future editions.

Endorsements of the Book Include:
Healthcare Information Technology Association
Healthcare Information Technology Stimulus Center

Editors, Proofreaders, and Reviewers of this Book include:
Laura Brenner, PhD; Laura Brenner Writing Services
Kellie Butkiewicz, PhD
Kelly J. Cooper, KJC Edits

Contents

Introduction

Health Care Information Technology (HCIT) is a unique field that continues to evolve every year. It consists of many components, has its own specific terminology, plays a part in many tangential fields, and brings together a variety of organizations through the use of various information systems. Perhaps most notably, HCIT includes various types of medical applications.

HCIT consists of both software and hardware components that follow the platforms of the networking development life cycle for medical applications, Electronic Medical Record (EMR) systems, medical systems, miscellaneous software, and various hardware components within the field. Some of the different types of organizations that use HCIT by way of Healthcare Information Systems—e.g., medical applications, EMR systems, and medical systems—include hospitals, urgent care centers, insurance companies, and private doctor's offices.

The field of HCIT is progressing rapidly. While this brings new awareness to the value of the field, it also creates a number of terminology mix-ups with other similar industries. Because of the unique lexicon of HCIT, one can quickly become overwhelmed by the new vocabulary and feel lost when attempting to understand the field-specific documents and other communications.

Here are some critical acronyms used within the industry. The following list includes definitions as well as some guidance on when and how each term should be properly used. More acronyms as well as other terms at the intersection of medicine and information technology and their definitions can be found at the end of the book, in the dictionary provided.

- Health Information Administration (HIA), when used in this field, should refer to office and administrative procedures of all health care practices.
- Healthcare Informatics, when used in this field, should refer to Medical Applications and Medical Software.
- Healthcare Information Technology (HCIT), the hardware and software focus, when used in this field, should refer to Healthcare Information Technology/Healthcare IT. It is sometimes abbreviated HC-IT or HIT.
- Health Information Management (HIM), when used in this field, should refer to HIM as well as the Certificate in Health Information Administration (CHIA), any Registered Health Information Administrator (RHIA), and Health (care) Information Management.
- Health Information Management, Healthcare Information Technology software and hardware, Health Informatics, and Health Administration, when used in this field, should refer to Health Information Systems toolkit (Healthcare Information Technology and/or Health Information Management techniques and scopes).

- IT, or *Information Technology*, when used in this field, should refer to *Healthcare Information Technology* (HIT, HCIT, or HC-IT) and includes mentions of computing technology like networking, hardware, and software.

Problems with the Industry

The Health Care Information Technology (HCIT) field has faced serious problems with regard to miscommunication, a lack of understanding, and unclear definitions with regard to where computer hardware and software fit in with all the data being transmitted in the field. Furthermore, the HCIT field has faced a possible problem with legislation; specifically with regard to how the U.S. Department of Health and Human Services will interpret what a "certified" Electronic Health Record (EHR) is. (This will be explored later in greater detail.)

Faced with these challenges, organizations and their research teams should conduct detailed research on HCIT and the applications they are attempting to implement—along with the hardware pieces they will be uniting with these applications.

For example, they may need to ask: How will new cell phone technology and various medical applications interact with the technology components of a larger program? Emphasis must be placed on the research that includes procedures and technologies that allow for developing, running, envisioning, and understanding a varied array of digital content, as well as how it affects individuals, groups, organizations, societies, and globally distributed systems.

Another point to consider is that any data is only part of a "knowledge life cycle" that advances from (1) data to (2) knowledge to (3) research. Thus, players in this field need to expect unexpected events and uncertainties in order to account for new technologies, services and applications. Some of these considerations include varieties of applications, heterogeneity of devices, network size and topology, networking technologies, and mobility patterns.

The Top-Down Model and Network Development Life Cycle for the World of Health Care Information Technology

THE TOP-DOWN MODEL AND NETWORK DEVELOPMENT LIFE CYCLE FOR HEALTH CARE INFORMATION TECHNOLOGY[1]	
Top-Down Model	Information Systems Development Process
Business	Strategic business planning Business processing
Applications	Systems development life cycle Systems analysis and design Application development life cycle
Data	Database analysis and design Database distribution analysis
Network	Network development life cycle Network analysis and design
Technology	Physical network design Network implementation Technology analysis

One should note that this chart presents an *ideal* description of the way that an HCIT system should be designed and implemented within the health care industry. In other words, developers and HCIT professionals should first examine the field from a bird's eye view before choosing specific applications and implementations to solve a particular problem or improve workflow.

Unfortunately, this does not describe the way that HCIT has been developed and implemented, in the past.

---

[1] Summers, 2011.

Rather than follow the "Top-Down" model outlined above, some organizations made the mistake of taking a "Bottom-Up" approach to HCIT—that is, software and hardware developed without any regard for the costs and timeliness of implementation, where they will ultimately be implemented, or how they will be integrated with existing systems or networks.

As a result, hospitals across the United States have been left with a number of problems as well as the logistical nightmare of implementations that may *not* have followed the top-down model. As of the time of this book's publication, a number of health care organizations were having difficulty collecting payments electronically as a result of HCIT issues. This lack of foresight and confusion has directly translated into an industry-wide loss of several billion dollars.

History of Computers

In order to understand the scope and context of the problems faced in the 21st century, we should first explore the history of computers as a whole and how they began to affect the world of health care.

It is amazing how computation evolved from using our own fingers and toes to count to the complex technology that the world possesses now. The oldest clue to the earliest form of a computer was the carvings of prime numbers into a bone, found sometime around 8500 BCE (Before the Common Era).

Sometime between 1000 BCE and 500 BCE, the abacus evolved. This instrument had movable beads whose positions changed in such a way that its user could enter numbers and perform mathematical computations.

The world's first mechanical calculator was created by Leonardo da Vinci in 1500. Then in 1642, Blaise Pascal's adding machine replaced Leonardo's basic calculator, moving computing forward again.

During the 19th century, English mathematician Charles Babbage introduced plans for a machine called the Babbage Difference Engine. Though it was designed to calculate numbers, it was able to print mathematical tables. Since Babbage was unable to construct the actual device, he received significant criticism. This challenged Babbage to address the limitations of his design. So he next developed plans for the Babbage Analytical Engine. This computing device would use punch cards as the control mechanism for calculations, a feature that would allow previously performed calculations to be used for future ones.

Soon Babbage met Ada Byron Lovelace, a woman who was passionate about mathematics. Lovelace saw new possibilities for the Analytical Machine, including the production of graphics and music. His project became a reality with her help. She documented how the device would calculate Bernoulli numbers. Lovelace subsequently was recognized for writing the world's first computer program. A computer language was even named after her by the U.S. Department of Defense in 1979.

Every computer that was developed built on the successes of previous ones. The first programmable computer arrived in 1943 named the Turing COLOSSUS. It was developed to decode German messages during World War II.

In 1946, ENIAC (Electronic Numerical Integrator And Computer), "The Giant Brain," became the first electronic digital computer developed by the U.S. Army during World War II.

Then in 1951, the U.S. Census Bureau became the first government agency to buy the first commercial computer built in the United States—the UNIVAC (UNIVersal Automatic Computer).

Soon people began connecting computers together, point-to-point, allowing them to communicate. This type of communication evolved into more and more complex capabilities that ultimately resulted in the creation of the original Internet in the late 1960s and early 1970s.

In 1977, computers were expanded to consumers with the release of the Apple computer. Soon after in 1981, the IBM Personal Computer (PC) for consumers was released even though IBM mainframes were already in use by government and corporations at that time.

The main protocol used to run the modern Internet, TCP/IP (Transmission Control Protocol/Internet Protocol), was created in the 1970s by the U.S Department of Defense. Meanwhile in 1980, Tim Berners-Lee developed the World Wide Web and CERN (the European Organization for Nuclear Research) released the first web server in 1991. The development of the web was the fundamental technology that popularized the Internet around the world.

Current computer technologies include word processing, games, email, maps, medical systems, data manipulation, and streaming data. Computers continue to evolve at a breakneck pace.[2]

Computers and Health Care Information Technology

As we have previously discussed, HCIT is the computer technology—consisting of both hardware and software—that is used within health care organizations.

The first computers intended for business use arrived on the market in the 1960s, and they replaced both the low-cost/low-performance drum memory devices and the high-cost/high-performance systems that used vacuum tubes (and later transistors) as memory.

---

[2] MerchantOS web site. "The History of the Computer."

Computer hardware and software started being used in wider numbers around 1975, when the first home computer, the Altair 8800, became popular. Though the term "medical application" was not yet in use, software and hardware components were already being used in the radiology field.

On November 8, 1895, Wilhelm Conrad Röntgen accidentally produced an image cast from his cathode ray generator (an Xray). This may have been the beginning of the discovery of the first medical applications, which would have consisted of computer hardware and images, but lacked coding.

The medical applications, computer software, and computer hardware in HCIT have evolved over the years and include the advancement of medical devices, hearing aids, medical imaging systems, remote patient monitoring and diagnostics, and medical alarm applications.

A suggested *workable* set of requirements for a medical application are as follows: First, that the application be paired with a medical device, hearing aid, medical imaging system (or remote patient monitoring and diagnostics and medical alarm applications), and second, that the top-down development life cycle is used to create the application's software.

Some medical applications use proprietary software; this depends on the organization's needs. Some medical applications are created by a software developer for a single organization.

Terminology Defined

Health Care Information Technology vs. Health Information Management

Two terms that often get mixed up are "Health Care Information Technology" (HCIT) and "Health Information Management" (HIM).

Health Care Information Technology is the application of information processing—which involves both hardware and software—to store, retrieve, and share health care information. HCIT allows for data and knowledge within the industry to be communicated to a number of agents, which greatly aids the decision-making process. HCIT also involves networking and building computer and communication systems to transmit this health care information. Likewise, HCIT involves the engineering of new information systems.[3]

HCIT's minimum components include a server to store data, a client computer with an operating system, and software that addresses each organization's unique needs. Most components of a medical application are installed and configured depending on the type of data that will be transmitted to and from them.

Health Information Management is the practice of maintaining and caring for health records via traditional and electronic means in health care facilities like hospitals and physician's offices, as well as health insurance companies, and other entities that provide health care or the maintenance of health records. Health informatics and HCIT are both a part of Health Information Management processes.[4]

---

[3] Wikipedia web site. "Health Information Management."
[4] Ibid.

Health Information Management also includes gathering data, analyzing it, and making it available to those who need it. Its ultimate objective is to enable the delivery of quality health care to the public.

EMR vs. EHR

EMR (Electronic Medical Record) and EHR (Electronic Health Record) are two terms that are often used interchangeably. They are interrelated, but there are a few distinctions between the two terms.

In his medical blog, Houston Neal, Marketing Director at Software Advice, clearly outlined the differences between EHR and EMR; he used the definitions recently drafted by National Alliance for Health Information Technology (NAHIT).

According to NAHIT's definitions, an **EMR** (Electronic Medical Record) is "the electronic record of health-related information on a per that is created, gathered, managed, and utilized by licensed clinicians and staff from *a single organization* involved in the person's health and care."

An **EHR** (Electronic Health Record) is the collective "electronic record of health-related information on an individual that is created and gathered cumulatively across *more than one* health care organization and is managed and consulted by licensed clinicians and staff involved in the individual's health and care."[5]

In more practical terms, an individual's record from a single organization is an EMR; an individual's record pieced together from more than one health care organization is an EHR. Under this definition, and because a single provider may create an EMR only through its own hardware and software systems, EMR is used more commonly and where appropriate.

---

[5] Neal, 2008.

Data and Medical Applications

Health Information Management involves managing different types of patient data, using Health Care Information Technology.

Data is defined as various types of information, usually formatted in a specific way.

In the health care field, the data used includes the <u>Patient's Information</u> (that is, *Name, Address, Social Security Number, and Medical Insurance Information*), and the <u>Patient's ID Number</u> (defined as the *MRN*, or *Medical Record Number*).

In the HCIT field, the protection of data is carried out through the use of *Usernames, Passwords, MRN,* and *Policies and Procedures.*

Let us first define these terms for clarity's sake:

<u>Usernames</u> and <u>Passwords</u> are unique sets of characters for the use of one specific person.

The National Committee on Vital and Health Statistics (NCVHS) defines an <u>MRN</u> (Medical Record Number) as a string of numbers and/or letters used in the process of identifying a patient. It further explains that each provider organization keeps and maintains a Master Patient Index (MPI), and the MRN is issued and maintained through this index.

The MRN, according to NCVHS, is also used to identify an individual and his or her medical record/information. The numbering system—plus the content and format of the MRN—is mostly specific to the particular organization.[6]

The <u>Policies and Procedures</u> vary from organization to organization, depending on the organization's needs. For example, HIPAA (the Health Insurance Portability and Accountability Act of 1996) is a law that all health care organizations have to follow. HIPAA now has standards and guidelines that must be met when dealing with HCIT.

For example, HIPAA sets certain guidelines with regard to health care computer security, due to the fact that systems and applications may vary widely in terms of how actively and efficaciously they prevent unauthorized users from accessing data.

Medical Applications are defined as unique applications installed on a client computer that have proven to be in compliance with all policies and procedures.

Additionally, a medical application is any computer program that is used within a health care organization. For example, it can include software that connects to medical devices, hearing aids, medical imaging systems, remote patient monitoring and diagnostics, or medical alarm applications.

---

[6] U.S. Department of Health and Human Services web site. "Understanding Health Information Privacy."

EHR Software

Readers should understand, first and foremost, the mechanics of modern (that is, electronic) patient data. In general, the field relies on the use of hardware and software that scan paper medical records and convert them into computer images. At this point, such images are saved in a health care provider's Electronic Health Record (EHR) software and stored on site. Typically, these images take the form of PDFs (which originally stood for "Portable Document Format" but which is now used as a noun to refer to a document in this format), an industry standard documentation format developed by the Adobe Systems company. As each image is scanned, these records become part of a larger virtual warehouse of health care data.

While the finer details of EHR software—including additional features, cost of purchase/implementation, and ease of use—vary from program to program, readers should note that they all work toward a common goal: scanning and securely storing images. At this phase, these medical records can be read by nearly any personal computer's default PDF viewer (typically, most use the commonly available Adobe Acrobat) and accessed with only a few mouse clicks.

EHR software also excels at providing users with easily manageable data. As the patient's medical records are scanned into the system, the software saves them in relevant folders and clinical categories. On the whole, these programs are affordable and high-quality.

The primary concern of this book is that this software *can*, however, vary widely in terms of how it complies with the provisions of HIPAA. Not all software is created equal, and any scanning and data storage software will need to be extensively tested by health care providers prior to final implementation in order to ensure absolute compliance, familiarity with use of the software, and compatibility with the program's users.

Readers will learn more about HIPAA and other important legislation in the "Legislation" chapter.

The Hardware and Software Focus of Health Care Information Technology

Combining hardware and software should be the most important focus of an implementation project of medical applications, EMR systems, and medical systems. Simply put, without software and hardware working together, there can be no medical software, medical applications, medical systems, or EMR systems.

As we already know, an EMR constitutes the electronic record of health-related information for an individual that is created, gathered, managed, and used by licensed clinicians and staff from a single organization who are involved in the individual's health and care. Once this information is gathered, it is then called *data*. The data is then input, manipulated, and stored on (or in) medical software and accessed by a medical device.

To further clarify, the definition of HCIT software includes the operating system—which is used to direct the operation of the computer—as well as any programs, data, and documentation that provides instructions on how to use those programs held by the computer's storage. The definition of hardware in this context is all-inclusive and defines the physical parts of a computer, as distinguished from the data it has or operates on.

For this reason, we see that the success of a provider's HCIT systems depends entirely on both components working together to achieve a common goal in the world of health care. An HCIT team cannot focus simply on software, or choose to solve a problem solely by upgrading hardware. It is the interplay between the two that results in productive workflow and superior care provided to patients.

Specific HCIT Hardware and Software

We turn to the academic world in order to better understand the number of components that are interrelated on the most basic level. Research compiled by Nick Benik and Dr. Griffin Weber, along with other industry peers, reveals that all of the following are essential hardware and software components of medical software, medical applications, medical systems, EMR systems, and implementations. Software and hardware for medical software, medical applications, medical systems, and or EMR systems include:

Hardware

- Desktop PCs
- Laptops
- Servers
- Tablets

Software

- Axis2 v1.1 web service (SOAP/REST messaging)
- Database Server 10g database
- Java 2 Standard Edition 6.0 version 16
- JBoss Application server version 4.2.2.GA
- Operating Systems
- Spring Web Framework 2.0
- Tablet PC Systems
- UX
- Xerces2 XML parser

Browser Requirements

- Internet Explorer 6 or 7, Firefox 2 or 3, or Safari 3

- JavaScript must be enabled

Server Requirements

- AJAX (asynchronous JavaScript and XML)
- Independent platform
- Proxy must be written for the type of server that is hosting it
- Server-side proxy
- Use of a proxy
- Web server that supports HTML, JavaScript, CSS, & GIF/JPG/PNG image files

Configuration of the Web Client

- Ability to be modified using any text editor
- Clear root directory
- Detailed documentation on each of the configuration settings
- New environment
- Standard JSON-style layout

Security Requirements

The security of medical software, medical systems, EMR systems, and medical applications relies on user ID/password combinations. Most EMR systems, medical applications, medical software, and medical systems implement basic security behaviors including:

Authentication: The requirement of at least a user name and a password for each user in order to access data.

Authorization: Users may only access categories that they are allowed to with the permission of a superior. This can be built into each user's account, allowing for different levels of authorization.

Confidentiality: Sensitive data must be encrypted by a computer algorithm in order to keep it private and secret.

Data Integrity: Data sent across the network cannot be modified or deleted by unauthorized users.

Legislation

Now that we have a better idea of the systems, software, and applications in place, the scope of the role that computers have in the health care industry, and the importance of maintaining a dual hardware and software focus, we can turn our attention to the way in which legislation dramatically affects the duties and importance of HCIT within the field.

The American Recovery and Reinvestment Act of 2009

Meaning & Use

The American Recovery and Reinvestment Act of 2009 (and known by its shortened acronym of ARRA) was signed into law by President Obama on February 17, 2009. In passing the act, the legislation placed a number of the president's agenda points into direct action. The president's technology agenda explains the goal of ARRA:

> *[To] Lower Health Care Costs by Investing in Electronic Information Technology Systems... [To] Use health information technology to lower the cost of healthcare... [To] Invest $10 billion a year over the next 5 years to move the U.S. healthcare system to broad adoption of standards-based electronic health information systems, including electronic health records.*[7]

In the final bill, $59 billion was earmarked for health care, with about $20 billion for EHR adoption. Obviously, many health care providers who are interested in EHR will want to know how to claim some part of this massive $20 billion allocation.

---

[7] US Innovation web site. "The Obama-Biden Plan."

First, $17 billion will be distributed in the form of incentives, distributed as increased Medicare and Medicaid payments. The incentives will start rolling out in 2011 and be paid over five years to physicians who can show "meaningful use" of an EHR system (what constitutes *meaningful use* will be defined later). Conversely, physicians who do not prove "meaningful use" will be reprimanded via lower Medicare payments. Hospital physicians will not be affected.

Those entitled to some portion of the stimulus money will also have to use a "certified" EHR system. As with the term "meaningful use," the definition of a "certified" system has not been defined by the government.

The maximum a provider can receive is $44,000 over a period of five years, paid either in a lump sum or through payments determined by the U.S. Department of Health and Human Services. Furthermore, and in order to be eligible for these funds, the physician must also use electronic prescribing in a meaningful way.

With respect to ARRA and the Health Information Technology for Economic and Clinical Health Act (the HITECH act, a subsection of ARRA), the stipulations detailed in these laws dovetail neatly with the focus of this book: HCIT hardware and software. The ARRA and HITECH acts involve requirements for EMR systems, medical applications, medical software, and medical system implementations.

Health Information Management Policy and Standards Committee

Better Known as the Health Information Technology Policy

While the details of "meaningful use" under ARRA are in need of clarification, the act does require that physicians demonstrate that EHR technology improves the quality of health care provided, including care coordination. He or she must also submit information on clinical quality measures as specified by the U.S. Department of Health and Human Services (HHS).

Under the provisions of ARRA, a Health Information Technology (HIT) Policy Committee formed under the auspices of the HHS will focus on development of a nationwide health information infrastructure; in pursuit of this goal, the committee will recommend standards, implementation specifications, and certification criteria.

It is clear that the timeline for implementing electronic health records to receive federal incentive payments will create demand for a variety of qualified professional services leading up to 2012 and beyond.

With respect to this book and for the purposes of clarity, the above policy may have been better named the "Health Information Management Policy" given the various definitions that are becoming standard.

Summary of ARRA Details for HCIT Implementation

- Acceleration of the construction of the National Health Information Network (NHIN)
- Creation of extension programs to facilitate regional adoption efforts
- Creation of grant and loan programs

- Development of educational programs to train clinicians in EHR use and to increase the number of health care IT professionals
- Provision of $40,000 in incentives (in 2011) for physicians to use EHRs
- Provision of funds to states to coordinate and promote interoperable EHRs

HITECH Defined

The Health Information Technology for Economic and Clinical Health Act (HITECH Act) was passed largely to create a pathway for the adoption of Electronic Medical Records; the act was part of ARRA and was signed into law by President Obama in 2009. A critical factor to understand the HITECH Act, with respect to HCIT's dual hardware and software focus, HITECH may have been better named "Health Information Management Economic and Clinical Health Act," due to its intent to work within the management of data. But the HCIT hardware and software focus is a major part of it.

According to HITECH, health care providers will be offered financial incentives in 2010 if they comply with the details of the act with regard to implementation and functionality of their EMRs. These financial incentives will be provided by the U.S. government in and or up to 2015, after which time fines may be assessed for non-compliance with the legislation.

Subtitle D of the HITECH Act addresses the privacy and security concerns that often go hand-in-hand with EMRs.

In particular, section 13410(d) of the HITECH Act states that there will be:

- A maximum penalty amount of $1.5 million for violations
- Four categories of violations
- Four corresponding tiers of penalty amounts

The main lesson a health care provider should take away from the HITECH Act is this: Improving the quality and scope of your HCIT now will translate into financial gain; whereas procrastination may carry a hefty sum in fines and other penalties.

HIPAA "Protected Health Information" Definition

HIPAA set up a variety of guidelines with regard to how Protected Health Information (PHI) may be shared or otherwise disclosed. In fact, the act contains a variety of titles that address these details. Title II of HIPAA, the Administrative Simplification provision—or in short, AS—assures that privacy is upheld within the health care industry. Perhaps most importantly, HIPAA allows national standards of electronic health care transactions to be endorsed by the HHS.

Primarily, the AS provision in Title II of HIPAA attempts to set certain guidelines, benchmarks, and other performance criteria that can be followed by America's employers, health care providers, and health insurance plans. A summary of these rules is as follows:

- The Enforcement Rule
- The Privacy Rule
- The Security Rule
- The Transactions and Code Sets Rule
- The Unique Identifiers Rule (National Provider Identifier)

HIPAA Exceptions to Protected Health Information

Readers should note that the guidelines established by HIPAA are not all-encompassing. Some exceptions *do* exist with regard to how the act affects PHI. For example:

• HIPAA does not apply to any information collected or maintained by an educational provider with regard to that entity's students. That is, data recorded about an individual collected and maintained as part of educational pursuit, which includes professional training, does not constitute PHI.

• HIPAA faces a number of exceptions under a variety of clauses within the Educational Rights and Privacy Act (20 USC). Specifically, there are a number of instances in which a patient's data may be accessed or shared with no obligation to inform the individual that such records were accessed or shared.

• When the "covered entity" is the employer, the guidelines do not apply. More simply, information that an employer personally collects from employees and maintains as part of his or her employment records specifically falls outside the purview of HIPAA.

With this in mind, let us take a look at what HIPAA defines specifically as Protected Health Information (PHI), as well as additional examples of what it is *not*.

The section of HIPAA entitled "the Privacy Rule" specifically creates a data category known as *De-identified Health Information*. In short, this is patient information that lacks *identifiers*, or any information that can connect the data back to the specific individual from whom it was collected.

Identifiers in PHI consist of all of the following:

- Date-based data
- Email IDs
- Fax details
- Fingerprints/voiceprints
- Geographic classifications that are smaller than a state (i.e., city or voting district information)
- Health plan beneficiary number(s)
- IP addresses
- License plate numbers
- PANs (Personal Account Numbers)
- Social Security Numbers
- URLs

If information is stripped of all of these identifiers, it no longer falls under the protection of HIPAA and can be safely disclosed. The health care provider does not have to worry about facing non-compliance-related penalties as a result of disclosing this data or using it for statistical purposes. Under HIPAA, data lacking any of the above bullet points has been found to have no danger of compromising the identity of individuals or the safety of their records.

In order to ensure full compliance under HIPAA, we recommend that any entity interested in de-identifying their health data consult a qualified statistician.

The Cost of HCIT and Legislative Noncompliance

Make no mistake, having HCIT systems noncompliant or failing to follow the requirements of the legislation described above can be absolutely toxic to a hospital's bottom line. Given that the field is so new and specialized and growing rapidly, it is hard to acquire the relevant experience. This chapter presents the reader with an inside look at the level of damage that noncompliant HCIT systems can cause.

The issue of being noncompliant may be not intentional. It could be due to a lack of knowledge due to the difficulty of keeping up with the rapid growth of the industry as well as the problem of providers being under the new constraints and deadlines.

Major Data Breaches

Health care providers have more to worry about than simply preventing employees from within the company from accessing data. In particular, significant and far-reaching breaches of medical data can be caused by poor information storage protocols or simply allowing employees to transport protected information to unsecure areas.

In October of 2010, one company that oversaw two separate health plans lost a flash drive containing the health records of more than 280,000 people. This information was not de-identified, and while the complete social security numbers of only four patients was stored on the drive, partial SSNs were used for more than 800 patients, along with personal information that identified hundreds of thousands of other individuals.

This breach was significant not simply because of the number of individuals compromised by the loss, but because the loss was entirely preventable. The company stated that the drive traveled to a variety of community health fairs. Such information should have been kept under lock and key at all times. Instead, the company facilitated the transport of this PHI to an environment that was not only unsecure but particularly hectic.

To make matters worse, the fact that the drive predominantly contained the information of Medicaid and Medicare recipients really caught the attention of the public as lower-income patients were placed at a greater risk of damage by identity theft they would find especially difficult to afford to fix.

The largest breach of patient data thus far occurred under similar circumstances.

In 2006, an employee of one health care administration transported a flash drive containing the health records of more than 2.5 million U.S. veterans to his home office; at some point, this data was stolen.

Breaches are far more numerous than one might suspect. For example, according to figures published by the Privacy Rights Clearinghouse, 184 separate breaches of medical data were reported in 2009 and 2010, which compromised the records of over 5 million individuals.

As mentioned, state guidelines may differ from federal guidelines with respect to penalties and the mandatory reporting of security breaches. Medicaid, for example, is jointly funded by the federal government and by each state, which adds another layer of complexity to a health care provider's responsibilities. For instance, while federal guidelines mandate that a company or health care provider must disclose a breach of PHI within 60 days, some states require that a breach be reported within 48 hours of discovery.

As for *who* must be notified, federal law requires that notification be provided to the individuals affected, the U.S. Secretary of Health and

Human Resources, media contacts—and of course, to the regulatory agencies in the state in which the breach occurred.[8]

The full scope of dealing with the aftermath of a security breach is far too complicated to describe in this book. Instead, the author ascribes to the notion that an ounce of prevention is worth a pound of cure. The absolute best way to avoid the headaches associated with breach-related notification guidelines, lawsuits, penalties, court defenses, and a host of other problems is simply to prevent the breaches from occurring in the first place.

It is critical for health care providers to note that security breaches can be a problem for *their* company or business model. It is for this reason that examination of the cost of such breaches is important to the industry as a whole. By doing this analysis, it can be understood just how prevalent these incidents have become.

The Total Cost of Data Breaches

An alarming report issued in 2009 by one medical research group revealed a shocking piece of information. Within the United States alone, the total cost of data breaches was an alarming $6 billion per year[10]; this number included legal fees and judgments, federal and state penalties, brand damage, investigation costs, notification costs, and other costs. Alternately, this institute determined that each individual record that is breached carried a cost.[9]

---

[8] Von Bergen, 2010.
[9] Ponemon L. "Annual study: Cost of a data breach."

The institute found all of the following to be true:

- Health care providers are stating that federal regulations—namely, HITECH—are attempting to improve the safety of patient records[10]
- Hospitals are possibly vulnerable to data breaches
- Hospitals should be protecting patient data
- Only a small percentage of health care organizations rely on security technology to prevent and detect data breach incidents
- Unintentional breaches of patient information are occurring frequently and often go unreported, which puts patients' privacy at risk

The most important piece of information to take away from the study is this: Hospitals should be in compliance with HITECH, HIPAA, and other regulations that can negatively impact their bottom line if not followed. While hospital officials and other health care providers tend to view complying with such regulation as "expensive," the $6 billion worth of costs incurred in 2009 speaks to the level of noncompliance that exists within the industry—not the costs of implementation.

---

[10] Nicastro, 2010.

Dangers of Noncompliance: A Look at Critical Industry Factors

Compliance with HIPAA is absolutely essential for any health care provider who wishes to avoid costly fines, lawsuits, undermining of patient confidence, negative press, or any combination thereof. We present a small and recent sampling of the fines and breaches encountered by several health care providers of varying sizes in a single state to clarify the scope and financial impact of these occurrences for each provider.

In February of 2009, a hospital was fined $25,000 for security violations. This occurred after a hospital employee was able to gain unauthorized access to the health records of a coworker's child.

In October of 2009, a hospital was fined $225,000 for similar violations of patient privacy; an unauthorized technician viewed the health records of nine patients, including those receiving psychiatric care and those who had been checked into the hospital's emergency room. After a police investigation, the technician revealed that the data accessed was used to open fraudulent cellular phone accounts.

In August of 2009, a health care provider was fined a total of $310,000 in fees after the medical records of nearly 600 patients were stolen. These paper records had been stored in a large, outdoor storage facility. Two different employees of the medical center each broke into this data storehouse and disclosed patient data on three separate occasions.

In October of 2009, an employee of one medical center was able to gain unauthorized access to the medical records of her sister-in-law. The center was found to be liable for these incidents and the hospital was assessed $60,000 in fees.

In March of 2009, another hospital was fined a total of $42,500 in fees after a member of the hospital staff posted the information regarding a patient's hospitalization on her personal web page, among other ethical breaches.

In July of 2009, a convalescence center was forced to pay more than $125,000 in patient privacy violation fees when a physical therapy aide gained unauthorized access to the medical records of five separate patients, which were then used for purposes of identity theft.

It should additionally be noted that, per HIPAA guidelines, these fines represent penalties issued by a state government. Many states across the nation have become increasingly vigilant about legal regulation and enforcement of violations after several high-profile security breaches. In particular, unauthorized parties accessed a number of medical records of Hollywood celebrities in 2008.

After the passage of more stringent laws that set mandatory fines for unauthorized data access, the first fine was issued to a major provider for more than $430,000; the stiff penalty was a result of the hospital's failure to secure the records of a famous person, whose data was accessed by a number of employees. [11]

Between the costs of HIPAA noncompliance and additional fees that may be assessed by state governments and regulatory agencies, very few organizations can justify the risk of unsecured data.

---

[11] Hennessy-Fiske, 2010.

Critical Information on How Outdated HCIT Affects Provider Revenue Cycles

All of these costs have so far focused solely on how having outdated or inadequate HCIT systems can affect a provider's bottom line with respect to fines and penalties. However, even if an organization is in the legal clear, outdated HCIT can still be an expensive proposition.

A health care provider's ability to receive timely payment is absolutely crucial to its continuing operations. This holds true in both office-based practices and primary care facilities. However, many health care providers are in need of a clear understanding of the effect that their HCIT systems have in terms of their financial bottom line. While the net effects of an outdated revenue cycle seem minor when judged by the cost created by each individual claim, these expenses can quickly spiral out of control. Some common problems are outlined below.

Insufficient Claims Process Monitoring

Providers need to have a management system that includes HCIT-compliant hardware and software in place to allow them to track a claim all the way through its lifecycle. This comes down to the strength of a provider's HCIT.

Additionally, a lack of automated alerts for denied claims by a payer for certain codes or procedures will result in a significant number of man hours being expended in order to research the problem. Rather than strain the human resources of the organization, a solid HCIT system coupled with a thorough workflow process can stop problems before they start.

A study from the University of California titled "Billing and Insurance-Related Administrative Costs: Burden to Health Care Providers" revealed that clerical follow-ups for rejected claims drain anywhere from 8 percent to 13 percent of a provider's annual revenue.[12] A critical factor here is that any organization wishing to reduce these costs will ensure its HCIT team is complete.

This team will be in the best position to provide a business process that allows for speedy and efficient follow-up to rejected claims, along with trouble-free archiving and documentation of all relevant error codes or denial messages. Proactive alerts provided by an HCIT system will allow these claims to be better understood and more easily and quickly rectified. This provides an immediate benefit to the provider's return on investment.

Outdated Payer Requirements

It is very easy to fall out of date with the rules and requirements of one's payer, due to the rapid changes in the industry. Worse yet, any claim that is merely resubmitted in the hopes of "working itself out" will often be rejected again, leading to the consumption of additional resources.

Often, this can occur when the structure of provider identification numbers changes. Before a claim can be resubmitted through the payer's system, it requires the provider's systems to be updated in order to support the change. Obviously, this requires time and money, and will delay payment for as long as one system remains out of date. During this time, the provider may discover varying degrees of cash flow problems, high numbers of claim rejections, and inflated administrative expenses.

Once again, having better HCIT in place can solve this problem before it starts. Qualified professionals will be in an excellent position to simplify the process of filing a claim. Moreover, such a team will be up-to-date with changes in a payer's policies or systems, and will be able to quickly

---

[12] Kahn, 2009.

modify the provider's systems in order to cut down on delays in the claims process.

Failure to Resubmit Rejected Claims

Simply put, the lack of follow-through on rejected claims will always correspond to a loss of revenue. In a perfect world, all providers would have the time and resources needed to resubmit every rejected claim, but this is simply not the case. Common barriers revolve around having inadequate data to allow the claim rejection to be fairly disputed.

A focused hardware and software HCIT team will be able to augment a provider's systems with up-to-date information and automated processes that identify where, when, and why claims were rejected. The team can also assist a provider by setting up automated appeal letters and automated re-filing of corrected claims.

Naturally, all of these steps will make it easier for a provider to recoup much of the revenue that could potentially be lost by any single rejected claim.

Outdated Patient Eligibility Verification

Virtually every U.S. health care provider is forced to write off bad debt as a result of patients who are ineligible for the care they ultimately end up receiving. Estimates reveal that one-fourth of all medical practices do not have systems in place that allow a provider to determine a patient's health care eligibility and co-pay amount prior to services being rendered. Another one-fourth have such systems in place, although they are not checked or otherwise accessed until the patient has already left the office.

Because revenue management is so critically tied to determining patient eligibility, solid HCIT software and hardware with a thorough workflow process allows a provider to easily and quickly determine if the practice will reasonably recover the expenses of the services rendered. Thus, improved IT systems will lead to increased revenue.

An up-to-date HCIT system with a thorough workflow process will automatically check patient eligibility and determine the amount of the patient's co-pay at the time he or she signs into the office. More sophisticated solutions may even be able to determine patient eligibility up to 24 hours in advance of the patient's visit. The bottom line is that good HCIT software and hardware with a solid workflow process can allow a provider to receive payment in full from patients and ensure that they are fairly and completely reimbursed by their payers.

Failure to Account for New Trends

In many hospitals, claims are processed one at a time. This is an unfortunate consequence of outdated IT and heavy administrative workloads. While in many cases, a small or moderate-sized hospital can get by with only a handful of administrators processing claims, they will nevertheless miss the big picture.

Solid HCIT allows a provider to ask the following question: What are the macro-level trends that affect our industry? Are we making the same kinds of errors repeatedly? Are we processing claims consistently and effectively?

In order to avoid loss of revenue due to repetition of the same errors or continued use of inefficient processes, an effective HCIT team could supply a provider with a number of workflow tools that can identify claims that are repeatedly denied, allowing the provider to repair or improve their processes. This will in turn improve the revenue cycle in both the short and the long term. After implementation, providers will be able to increase the acceptance rate of first-time claims and streamline their submission process.

Again, all of the HCIT deficiencies outlined above will definitely create a loss of revenue, sap internal resources, and could lead to poor management. Once again, all are problems that can be addressed through the efforts of a team of HCIT professionals who are used to assisting hospitals and other care providers.

The best teams will have a history of implementing payer-specific claims, editing solutions, and automating the verification of a patient's eligibility. Likewise, the team should have cutting-edge alert monitoring and auditing tools, in addition to software solutions that will allow a provider to correct claims online rather than on paper.

With such help, the time and resources freed up by the HCIT team will allow hospital or practice administrators to maximize their ability to collect outstanding debts and prevent losses of revenue before they are allowed to become reoccurring issues.

Commonalities among HCIT Problems While Implementing Medical Application, EMR systems, and/or Medical Systems

In general, each of these incidents—and indeed, most Information Technology problems an organization is likely to encounter as they provide health care—may be traced to one or more of the following possibilities:

- A lack of continuous IT project training
- A lack of knowledge about how software and hardware will affect the provider's bottom line
- A lack of research into where potential problems may occur in the implementation process, or areas where patient confidentiality and data security may become a factor

Because an experienced HCIT team is crucial to solving these problems, this book will address the issues related to finding, hiring, and utilizing such a team, as well as a number of related financial and logistical concerns.

Solving Problems with an HCIT Team

The HIM/HCIT field demands a high level of understanding before organizations can begin to take advantage of its opportunities and function within its changing guidelines and by-laws.

As a result, the demand for outside consultants and contractors continues to grow. These third parties can help health care providers by (1) assisting them in preparing for the demands of the HIM/HCIT; and/or (2) helping them assist other organizations once they have met their HCIT goals.

When selecting such consultants or organizations, one should ensure that they have direct access to a number of industry professionals and that they have a proven track record of performing HCIT work within the field of health care.

Further Industry Needs for "Certified and Educated" Professionals for Medical Systems Implementation

Certified, educated, and experienced HCIT contractors offer a variety of additional benefits to health care providers. In particular, these HCIT professionals can provide physicians and health care organizations with the following benefits:

- Consistent Training and Continuing education

  - Focuses on the Hardware and Software requirements of the EMR and HIPAA stimulus package

  - Provides company staff with essential HCIT knowledge

- Implementation
  - Assists healthcare providers to access the $20 billion of recent federal funds created through ARRA
  - Creates a roadmap to a successful EMR implementation

Critical thoughts of the industry about the ARRA Preparedness and Sustainability

Naturally, the $20 billion federal investment into ARRA has opened the door for a variety of new jobs, and many providers are understandably eager to receive a portion of those funds.

However, while the American Recovery and Reinvestment Act offers a substantial amount of financial incentives to health care providers who adopt EMRs and strengthen their IT, there are two reoccurring questions within the industry. First, are health care providers doing enough to secure those funds? And second, of those that are improving their systems, how many are going to be sustainable once ARRA is no longer offering incentive dollars?

A study by one of the largest health care management consulting firms in the United States was conducted to assess exactly these questions.

Among the study's findings were the following:

- Fifteen percent of respondents have operational Health Information Exchanges (HIEs). Approximately 60 percent have HIE plans in development and more than 20 percent are in the pre-planning stages.

- Forty-five percent of respondents have not applied for any federal or local grants, which could help them with HIEs and eventually achieving meaningful use.

- Most health care organizations have included HCIT spending into their financial plans for the coming years to help support patient care, clinical quality, and safety as part of their annual spending, tactical planning, and strategic multi-year plans.

- Quality reporting is the biggest concern among 73 percent of respondents.

- More than 40 percent of respondents have plans to enhance their physician and patient portals, which are crucial to the development of a sound and secure infrastructure at any health care organization.

- Most health care organizations (more than 80 percent) will either maintain or increase their HCIT investments if it is determined that they meet the *meaningful use* definition necessary to receive incentive payments. [13]

In addition, the report warned that implementation is no easy matter; it requires the input of qualified professionals within the industry and a significant amount of capital and administrative labor in order to be successful.

The logical extension of the report's findings is this: Within the next five years, health care providers can expect the demand for qualified HCIT professionals to be filled, and the number of consultants and services on the market that will help organizations meet the demands of ARRA will increase.

Implementation and Compliance

Successful implementation within one's organization should include a team of professionals from the fields of business planning management,

---

[13] Hartman, 2010.

HCIT service management, HCIT compliance, software change management, deployment and release management, and HCIT portfolio management. Your agency should create solutions that ensure that your requests, changes, and releases are consistently captured, viewed, and tracked across your entire HCIT organization. Your agency should thoroughly define and manage processes, adapt to changing circumstances, and release management solutions that can help gain HCIT compliance.

Determining Your Organization's Complete Platform &

Business Planning

Just as many successful companies need a business plan to guide their operations; it would be prudent for your HCIT team to create a business plan for implementation. In essence, having a business plan prior to beginning implementation allows you to put theory into practice.

Historically, here are just some of the reasons why successful companies make a solid business plan for medical applications, EMR systems, medical systems, and the backbone of their organization:

• A business plan helps the management team define the constraints in which they work. It prompts a team to analyze its project or the problem at hand critically and in an even-handed manner. Therefore, the business plan not only creates a set of goals, but ensures that efforts are focused towards achieving *realistic* goals. It also standardizes the basis under which evaluation of project effectiveness will occur.

• A good business plan always reveals shortcomings or omissions inherent in a plan. A risk calculated and projected in a business plan allows a team to more easily and quickly adapt to a problem when and if it occurs.

- Business plans are historically a company's go-to method of providing lenders, banks, investors, and employees with an understanding of why a business does what it does. A great plan keeps employees motivated and investment capital available. Even when not required to obtain a loan, a business plan always increases a company's chance of obtaining one.

Within the world of HCIT, a business plan for implementation should take into consideration all deadlines that affect a project. In addition, it should outline the responsibilities of each individual, project organization, and department involved.

In short, the organization, HCIT director, and project manager must have a clear idea of how the effort will influence every aspect of the larger business. Therefore, the plan will include all of the following at a bare minimum:

- A plan to monitor implementation and progress
- Management team summary
1. List of key personnel
2. Relevant business experience and expertise

- Organizational structure
- Overall business objectives
- Tasks required to attain the objectives
- Timeline for HCIT implementation

During a presentation to your immediate directors, be sure to demonstrate a strong management team, which can enhance your business plan by showing that you can apply your good ideas and theory in the real world. The importance of an experienced, effective management team *cannot* be understated.

Only through a clearly written and thoughtfully drafted implementation plan will your project be a success. To ignore this step is to throw caution to the wind, and will undoubtedly waste time and resources. Plan ahead and attempt to account for all contingencies.

Critical Compliance Factors

One thing that health care organizations may need to realize is that most compliance requirements can be mandatory. However, the manner of compliance is more crucial than a mere pass-or-fail of the HIPAA guidelines.

How compliance is achieved can determine an organization's ability to bill, collect, and input data. In certain cases, it may even affect an organization's financial and operational performance.

The following are guidelines that will help in successful implementation and compliance with regard to medical applications, EMR systems, and medical systems:

Awareness of Rules
Misinformation and misunderstanding surround the terminology, definitions, policies, transactions, and rules that govern the HCIT field. Thus, awareness of federal, state, and company-level rules and regulations is very important to successful implementation and legal compliance.

Change Leadership and Business Process Reengineering
There will always be resistance to change if it is viewed as a disruption to the customary way of doing things. However, if change is viewed as an expansion or advancement, it will be welcomed and even embraced.

Need for Urgency
There is an urgent need to comply and implement. The more an organization delays, the more the task will seem insurmountable to those charged with implementation.

Evaluation of All Systems and Processes

Gap analyses can be conducted to help develop a roadmap for making decisions regarding remediating, upgrading, replacing, or outsourcing systems and processes. Since it can be cost prohibitive to remediate legacy systems for some health care organizations, replacement of noncompliant systems could be the way to achieve compliance and business continuity.

Selection of Systems

To reduce implementation time, the number of interfaces, risk, and total cost of ownership (TCO), the strategy for health care organizations should be focused on selecting systems that provide interoperability and complete integration.

Evaluation of EMR Implementation Options

The use of an EMR system is particularly important in order for hospitals to obtain the full benefits of automated clinical documentation. The adoption of EMRs is a drastic operational change, especially for physicians. It can take anywhere from three to nine months on average for clinicians to adapt and recover from the loss of productivity that normally accompanies EMR implementation. If the EMR system is not carefully selected and properly implemented, lost physician productivity (25 percent to 40 percent on average) may never be recovered.

Obtaining the Right Tools

It is beneficial to talk with software vendors and learn who they are partnered with in order to implement coding and auto-coding. With the complexity and number of codes, manual coding is not realistic in most cases.

Value of Training

Training is consistently cited as a top critical success factor, and the number of staff members who need training is normally underestimated. The level of training needed within an organization will vary, but it is absolutely vital to provide training to key members at all levels.

Your Stimulus Team: An Overview

ARRA has stated within its stipulations that each organization should have an "EMR and HIPAA Economic Stimulus Team." An organization's stimulus team should consist of a trainer with a strong educational background and over 10 years' worth of training/teaching experience in an adult environment, specifically in the high technology arena.

Likewise, the team should include individuals who hold current certifications and at least a bachelor's degree in Information Technology. The team should have organizational and technical training experience that allows them to prove their ability to identify problems, analyze possible solutions, and determine the best course of action—all of which ensure that the organization's objectives will be successfully met.

Additional criteria for your organization's stimulus team include:

• Demonstration of familiarity in working with hardware and a variety of secure networks across several agencies and locations

• Demonstration of the ability to, as an effective trainer, deliver clear, concise, and engaging technology training for group and individual audiences

• Demonstration of the ability to collect, input, and report data to maintain records

• Demonstration of the ability to create and comply with a project plan, timeline, and budget

• The ability to function effectively both as an independent trainer and as an integrated team member

• The ability to solve problems creatively and effectively.

Training for the HCIT field has been a major challenge; historically, it has been difficult to find properly trained professionals. Since the passage of HITECH, HIPAA, and ARRA, many employers have been attempting to hire for positions necessary to ensure HCIT system security and legislative compliance. However, many employers are also seeking knowledge and training with regard to figuring out how to design the position and find the right candidate. Employers need to understand the requirements of each position and the skills needed to do the job. In addition, they must ensure that the professionals they hire have not only the proper training, but extensive knowledge about the position they are seeking to fill.

In today's rapidly expanding HCIT field, aspiring health care and information technology workers will require training, retraining, and skills upgrades to succeed in the HCIT workplace.

Hiring for Key Positions

Each critical member of an HCIT team should have every one of the following skills, experience, and knowledge before attempting any project that could compromise patient data:

- Experience with customer service
- Experience with medical records
- Experience with medical software systems
- Familiarity with Information Technology
- Familiarity with patient care
- Project management skills
- Work experience in a digital health care environment

The following guidelines for the <u>minimum</u> level of experience an organization should look for in an HCIT director and or stimulus team directors.

Qualifications:

- A strong customer service background
- An Information Technology background
- Bachelor's degree in a related field of study
- Comfort with a variety of software programs

- Experience as an IT director in a medical application environment; a minimum of five (5) years of relevant experience in IT communications and/or telecommunications
- Experience with "Go Live" situations
- Experience with implementation of medical applications
- Firsthand knowledge of working in a digital health care environment
- Good interpersonal relations; ability to meet deadlines; a self-described self-starter
- History of managing multiple projects concurrently
- Interpersonal and professional competencies, including continuing professional education and certification
- Medical record familiarity
- Medical software system familiarity
- Proven IT knowledge, skills, and abilities
- Proven project management skills
- Skills related to news gathering, writing/editing, electronic communications publishing, and web site content development
- Understanding of patient care

Principal Suggested Responsibilities of an HCIT Analyst/Stimulus Team Member and Suggested Required Experience

While the HCIT director should have the autonomy to choose his or her own team of hires and contractors necessary to complete a particular project, health care administrators often find it valuable to know who is responsible for what duties within their HCIT team. Beyond the HCIT director, the majority of HCIT teams and EMR stimulus teams consist of the following key members:

Business Analyst/Trainer

- Collects data to maintain records
- Inputs and reports data to maintain records

- Conducts training
- Works with staff to ensure that stored data is protected by adequate access restrictions

Client/Server Support Analyst/Trainer

- Collects, inputs, and reports data to maintain records
- Conducts training on network resources
- Implements security user accounts on new and existing servers
- Installs network connections
- Performs functions in server troubleshooting/client problems using remote desktop support

Program Coordinator

- Collects, inputs, and reports data to maintain records
- Communicates clearly and effectively with customers and staff
- Documents, tracks, and monitors problems to ensure timely resolution
- Draws from feedback and makes quality improvements in workshop delivery and content
- Implements secure user accounts on new and existing servers
- Manipulates data via the relevant operating systems and applications
- Solves problems creatively; effectively performs technical troubleshooting on site
- Works with hardware and a variety of secure networks across several agencies and locations
- Works with staff to ensure that stored data is protected by adequate access restrictions

Network Systems Analyst

- Performs functions in server troubleshooting/client problems via remote desktop support
- Performs functions in solutions design and software implementation
- Performs server and active directory administration
- Performs technical support for printers, networks, and software installations
- Performs technical support for software application issues
- Performs Tier II desktop support as a desktop technician
- Performs troubleshooting on desktop operating systems, and desktop applications
- Serves as network support analyst, providing an interface between system users and the technical support group with regard to troubleshooting

- Solves problems creatively; effectively performs technical troubleshooting on site

Systems Support Specialist

- Re-images systems as necessary
- Teaches adult learners desktop software applications
- Teaches in a multicultural environment while demonstrating superior customer service skills
- Trains staff on operating systems, applications, and computer repair
- Trains students on basic computer skills and basic computer troubleshooting skills
- Troubleshoots laptops, desktops, and PDAs
- Uses the remote desktop method to assist and troubleshoot software issues
- Works with hardware and a variety of secure networks across several agencies and locations
- Works with staff to ensure that stored data is protected by adequate access restrictions

Computer Programmer

- Creates user groups and user case workflows
- Designs, develops, and implements web sites
- Provides solutions for design and software implementation issues
- Troubleshoots, debugs, and implements software code

Application Analyst

- Assists with overall project management
- Conducts training on billing software for surrounding hospitals
- Performs scanning tasks

Help Desk/Customer Service Rep

- Communicates clearly and effectively with customers and staff
- Performs technical support on printers, networks, and software installations
- Performs technical support for software application issues

Nursing

- Communicates patients' questions, complaints, problems, and concerns to appropriate staff members
- Explains policies and procedures to patients and refers them to the proper departments
- Patient care

Introducing New Medical Applications in HCIT

There are various medical applications that can be used within your health care organization. However, your stimulus team needs to evaluate your organization's needs first and ensure that security is kept as a primary goal throughout any implementation of HCIT. Your applications should not run the risk of being accessible to hackers or competing organizations.

To comply with HIPAA, you (the medical organization) should include a confidentiality agreement between your company and the HCIT contractors during the implementation stage of your proprietary systems. This can simply be a part of your EHR stipulations.

What follows is a sample agreement:

The Collaboratee agrees to keep all of the Collaborator's business secrets confidential at all times. Collaborator's business secrets include any information regarding the Collaborator's customers, supplies, finances, research, development, manufacturing processes, or any other technical or business information.

The Collaboratee agrees not to make any unauthorized copies of any of the Collaborator's business secrets or information without Collaborator's consent, nor to remove any of Collaborator's business secrets or information from the Collaborator's facilities.

WHEREAS, Collaborator wishes to ensure that the confidential and proprietary information is protected from disclosure and only used by the Collaboratee for the purpose of evaluating and/or creating, developing, and designing and or accepting a collaboration project.

For this business purpose, the Collaboratee shall not use any ideas, information, health care certifications, employees, classes, companies, business, documents, contacts, computer software programs, corporate operations procedures, marketing plans and methods, customer lists, prospective client lists, (regardless of whether such lists have been distilled or tailored for the specific use of the Disclosing Party), for its sole purpose.

In addition, Collaboratee agrees that all information relative to carriers and any of the companies that are the primary source for the products of Collaborator are confidential and are not to be used by Collaboratee, unless Collaboratee has been given permission in writing by Collaborator to offer the products, only for joint purpose of this business relationship. This includes all information disclosed in oral, written, graphic, photographic, recorded, diagrammed, digital, electronic, or any other form by one party to the other, as well as the content of this agreement and the content of any and all discussions between the parties related to this agreement or otherwise;

WHEREAS, Collaborator wishes to ensure that upon completion of the review of the potential business relationship or termination of discussions between the parties, and/or termination of creating or developing permitted business purpose, and designing the Collaborator's collaboration project, that the confidential and proprietary information is returned to the Collaborator and/or not disclosed, or used for any purpose, at any time, by the Collaboratee. For the purpose of this business agreement and business-to-business relationship, all work performed, done, completed, requested to be completed, or created, and any and all other works, copyrights, exclusive rights, related rights, neighboring rights, works subject to copyright, exclusive rights granted by copyright, moral rights, right to be credited for the work, and copyright as property right is/are owned wholly, legally, solely, rights of, and created by (your company name).

Collaboratee to this agreement agrees not to compete, either directly or indirectly, with the business ideas, supplies, finances, research, development, manufacturing processes, or any other technical or business information of the (your company name) and affiliates.

Collaboratee agrees that "not to compete" means not to engage in any manner in a business or activity similar to the business ideas, supplies, finances, research, development, manufacturing processes, or any other technical or business information of the (your company) and affiliates.

The Collaboration term is defined for the purpose of this agreement as project thoughts and communication. There are no payment terms attached to this agreement.

If this agreement is violated, (your company name) and affiliates will be entitled to an injunction to prevent such competition, without the need for the buyer to post any bond. In addition, (your company name) and affiliates will be entitled to any other legal relief.

Implementation Costs

As previously discussed, any funds dedicated to increasing the quality and security of a health care provider's HCIT systems—or creating a new electronic system where one did not previously exist—is money well spent if it allows the company to avoid a $100 million lawsuit. Nevertheless, many smaller providers are concerned that they lack the budget or staff needed to build a secure system of medical records. As a result, the need for adequate HCIT systems continues to go unmet.

The following charts present a sample of the costs associated with implementing and maintaining a system of medical records, both in terms of the implementation cost per year and the tools needed to accomplish such a goal.

Small Project Cost Per Year

Staff	Budget	Facilities/ Other Resources	Budget
Data staff	$9,000	Rent	$6,000
Administrative staff	$9,000	Utilities	$6,000
Hardware staff	$10,000		
Director	$13,333	Equipment	$30,000
Medical applications (Software staff)	$10,000		
Design developer	$10,000	Travel	$3,520
Editorial staff	$9,000		
Accounting and bookkeeping staff	$3,000	Other	
Legal fees and staff	$3,000	Supplies	$12,000
		Publication/ Documentation/ Dissemination	$6,000
Benefits		Other Consultant Services	$6,000
Insurance	$5,000	Other Computer Services	$9,000
Training	$10,000		
		TOTAL	**$169,853**

Medium Project Cost Per Year

Staff	Budget	Software and Hardware	Budget
Data staff (1.5)	$50,000	Rent	$12,000
Administrative staff (1.5)	$50,000	Supplies	$64,000
Dell staff (2)	$50,000	Utilities	$10,000
Director (1)	$60,000		
Clinical Works (1.5)	$60,000	**Benefits for All Staff**	
Design Developer (1.5)	$60,000	Insurance	$50,000
Editorial staff (1.5)	$50,000	Training	$50,000
Accountant and booker staff (contract)	$6,000		
Legal fees and staff (contract)	$6,000	**TOTAL BUDGET**	**$578,000**

Large Project Cost Per Year and Budget Justification

Line Items	FT Equivalent Person-Months	Total Salary Per Year
Senior Project Personnel Salaries & Wages		
Director		$120,000
Administrative & Clerical Salaries & Wages		
i. Data staff (3)		$120,000
ii. Administrative staff (3)		$100,000
iii. Hardware staff (2)		$100,000
iv. Software staff (2)		$100,000
v. Design Developer (4)		$100,000
vi. Editorial staff (3)		$150,000
Accountant & booker staff, contract		$100,000
Legal fees and staff (contract)		$100,000
Fringe Benefits		
Insurance		$100,000
Training		$200,000
Equipment		
Travel		
Participant Support		
Other Direct Costs		
Materials and supplies		$100,000
Total Direct Costs		**$1,390,000**
Indirect Costs (rent and utilities)		$192,000
Total Direct and Indirect Costs		**$1,582,000**
Amount of This Request		**$1,582,000**
Cost Sharing		

Equipment Request for Implementation

Equipment	Budget

Software
   Cell Phone Applications
   Dreamweaver
   PHP Tools
   Visual Studio
	$10,000

Supplies
   Miscellaneous Supplies
   Paper
   Printer
	$12,000

Hardware
   2-Terabyte Drives
   8 Gigs of Ram
   Cell Phones
   Desktop PCs
   Laptops
   Monitors
   Quad Processor
   Servers
   White Board
   Wireless Devices
   Wireless Tools
	$20,000

TOTAL	**$42,000**

Final Thoughts

Hospitals are faced with the monumental tasks (albeit incentivized by several million dollars freed up through ARRA) of safeguarding patient information in a digital era, ensuring that they comply with numerous pieces of legislation, and integrating new technological solutions that will—in theory—allow them to provide better care to the patients in their charge.

This, however, is a job they cannot do alone. Doctors and nurses cannot be expected to become HCIT experts any more than HCIT experts can be trusted to perform surgery.

The effectiveness of the modern hospital will almost always go hand-in-hand with the effectiveness of its HCIT department. It is as essential to providing good care as the skills of the physicians, administrators, and nursing staff. Unfortunately, because HCIT happens behind the scenes, it is easy to marginalize the worth of what an IT team can provide to the modern hospital. As the saying goes, "out of sight, out of mind."

The fines stretching into the hundreds of thousands of dollars per major data breach speak volumes about the dangers of the laissez faire approach, as do the projected costs of lost manpower and disruptions to a health care provider's revenue cycle.

Today, the necessity of effective HCIT practices, and the need for these practices to be HIPAA-compliant, is more urgent than ever. The public and their legislators have spoken quite clearly about the need for safer, more fully interconnected, and more sophisticated electronic health records, and it falls on the shoulders of caregivers across the nation to deliver.

The modern hospital needs an experienced, skilled team of HCIT workers—each of whom is assembled and evaluated under an equally skilled director. It is the hope of this author that modern medicine will continue to enthusiastically welcome these professionals into its hospitals and care centers as vital and essential facilitators of the healing process.

Advice and Information

Author/Expert: Kellie Butkiewicz, PhD

Short Bio of Author/Expert:
Kellie Butkiewicz is a practicing school psychologist, and adjunct faculty member at Antioch University in Santa Barbara, CA.

Topic: Implementing HCIT within a Behavioral Health Clinical Setting

Issue:

The same issues that face implementing HCIT within the medical setting apply to the behavioral health arena. Like medical records, behavioral health care records are of the utmost confidentiality, and compliance with HIPAA is an absolute necessity when enacting new HCIT practices.

A significant issue facing mental health care practitioners in a private clinical setting is medical billing through consumers' insurance providers. Because of the complexity of billing, and subsequently the common difficulty health care providers face with having claims paid out upon initial submission of a claim, many mental health care providers in private practice are unwilling, or unable, to accept insurance as a form of payment. This is a serious issue for both providers and consumers of mental health care, resulting in a lack of quality care for consumers and financial strain for providers who do not have the time resources, or expertise, to efficiently bill for services.

Author/Expert Advice:

Training and software is needed within the mental health care field in order to bridge the gap between medical and behavioral health practices in terms of implementing HCIT compatible with HIPAA, as well as legislative requirements.

Health Care Information Technology

Dictionary

Below is a list of important definitions for health care technology professionals and those wishing to better understand and implement the provisions of the American Recovery and Reinvestment Act (ARRA) of 2009, the Health Insurance Portability and Accountability Act (HIPAA) of 1996, and the Health Information Technology for Economic and Clinical Health Act (HITECH) of 2009.

ADLs. The *activities of daily living*, i.e., those things we normally do to take care of ourselves, such as feeding, grooming, bathing, etc.[14] These are often used as measurements for a patient's functional status.

Applications Analysis. Support given to a certain application which may entail programming, system administration, problem analysis and diagnosis, finding the root cause of the problem, and solving the problem. Typically, "applications analysis" includes supporting custom applications programmed in a variety of programming languages and using a variety of database systems, middleware systems, and the like. It is a form of third-level line technical support.[15]

ARRA refers to the *American Recovery and Reinvestment Act of 2009*.

AS refers to the *Administrative Simplification* provisions in Title II of HIPAA, which require the establishment of national standards for electronic health care transactions and national identifiers for providers, health insurance plans, and employers.

---

[14] Wikipedia, "Certified Nursing Assistant."

[15] Wikipedia web site. "Application Analyst."

Authenticate. Allow access with the minimum requirement of having the user supply a username and a password.

Authorization. Allowing a user to access only categories of information allowed by permission of a supervisor or other superior.

Browser. Program used for accessing information on a network such as the World Wide Web.

Business Systems. Methodical procedures or processes used as delivery mechanisms for providing specific goods or services to customers in a well-defined market.[16]

Cell Phone. Hand-held mobile radiotelephone for use in an area divided into small sections, each with its own short-range transmitter/receiver.[17]

Cell Technician. Carries out proper fault diagnosis to improve the quality of the cell phone; carries out repairs on mobile phones to improve the phones' productivity. The main services offered by a cell phone technician are making repairs, keeping customers informed about services provided by the company (including warranties and after-sales services), and providing advice and recommendations about phones.[18]

Certified Nurse Aide/Patient Care Assistant. Person who assists individuals with health care needs (often called "patients," "clients," or "service users") with activities of daily living (ADLs). He or she also provides bedside care—including basic nursing procedures—all under the supervision of a Registered Nurse (RN) or Licensed Practical Nurse (LPN).[19]

---

[16] Business Dictionary web site. "Business System."

[17] Thefreedictionary.com web site. "Cellphone."

[18] Muchira, 2011.

[19] Wikipedia web site. "Certified Nursing Assistant."

CHIA. *Certificate in Health Information Administration*, necessary to become an **RHIA**.

CMS. *The Centers for Medicare and Medicaid Services.*

Confidentiality. Sensitive data must be encrypted.

CPT. *Current Procedural Terminology* is a registered trademark of the American Medical Association; it is a coding system for medical procedures in which numbers are assigned to the tasks and services that a medical practitioner might provide to a patient, including medical, surgical and diagnostic services; it allows for comparability in billing, pricing, and utilization review.[20]

CPT codes. Coding system for medical procedures that allows for comparability in billing, pricing, and utilization review.[21]

Customer Service. Service provided to a paying or nonpaying customer or client of any business.

Data Integrity. The assurance that data cannot be modified by an unauthorized user, the process, and/or means of transportation.

Digital Health Care Environment (DHE). A form of Electronic Health Recording (EHR). A DHE is a more secure environment which demands both advanced encryption and authentication processes for the users, thereby securing client information.

EHR (Electronic Health Record). The aggregate electronic record of health-related information on an individual that is created and gathered cumulatively across more than one health care organization and is

---

[20] Thefreedictionary.com web site. "CPT Codes."

[21] Thefreedictionary.com web site. "CPT Codes."

managed and used by licensed clinicians and staff involved in the individual's health and care.[22]

EMR (Electronic Medical Record). The electronic record of health-related information on an individual that is created, gathered, managed, and used by licensed clinicians and staff from a single organization who are involved in the individual's health and care.[23]

Hardware. An all-inclusive term for the physical parts of a computer, as distinguished from the data it has or operates on.[24]

HCIT. Abbreviation for *Healthcare Information Technology*, the hardware and software focus, and is sometimes referred to as **Healthcare IT** and **HIT**

HCPC Codes (Healthcare Common Procedure Coding). System of letter and number codes designated for procedures, supplies, medications, and equipment that are used for pricing and billing and are based on **CPT** codes.[25]

Health Care Information Management. Management of all patient data within a health care facility.

Health Care Information Technology. Support and/or management of the hardware and software in a health care facility.[26]

Health Information Management, Healthcare Information Technology software and hardware, Health Informatics, and Health Administration, when used in this field, should refer to the *Health Information Systems*

---

[22] Neal, 2008.

[23] Ibid.

[24] Open Projects web site. "Computer Hardware Definition."

[25] Cahaba Government Benefits Administrators web site. "Glossary of Definitions: HCPCS code."

[26] Ahima web site. "Health Information Careers: Glossary of Terms."

toolkit (Healthcare Information Technology and/or Health Information Management techniques and scopes).

Health Information Privacy. The Office for Civil Rights enforces each of the following: the HIPAA Privacy Rule, which protects the privacy of individually identifiable health information; the HIPAA Security Rule, which sets national standards for the security of electronic protected health information; and the confidentiality provisions of the Patient Safety Rule, which protects identifiable information from being used to analyze patient safety events and improves patient safety.[27]

Healthcare Informatics, when used in this field, should refer to medical applications and medical software.

Hearing Aids. Electro-acoustic devices, which usually fit in or behind the wearer's ears and are designed to increase and adjust sound for the wearer.[28]

HHS refers to the *U.S. Department of Health and Human Services*.

HIA. *Health Information Administration*, in this context, should refer to the office and administrative procedures of all health care practices.

HIE. A *Health Information Exchange*.

HIM. *Health Information Management*, sometimes written as *Healthcare Information Management*.

HIPAA. *The Health Insurance Portability and Accountability Act* (HIPAA) was enacted by the U.S. Congress in 1996. It was originally sponsored by Sen. Edward Kennedy (D-Mass.) and Sen. Nancy

---

[27] U.S. Department of Health and Human Services web site. "Understanding Health Information Privacy."

[28] Wikipedia web site. "Hearing Aid."

Kassebaum (R-Kan.). According to the Centers for Medicare and Medicaid Services (CMS) website, Title I of HIPAA protects health insurance coverage for workers and their families when they change or lose their jobs. Title II of HIPAA, known as the Administrative Simplification (AS) provisions, requires the establishment of national standards for electronic health care transactions and national identifiers for providers, health insurance plans, and employers.[29]

HIT. *Healthcare Information Technology*, the hardware and software focus, it is sometimes referred to as **Healthcare IT** and **HCIT**.

HITECH or **HITECH Act** refers to the *Health Information Technology for Economic and Clinical Health Act of 2009* (a subsection of ARRA).

Home Healthcare Aide. Trained and certified healthcare worker who provides assistance to a patient in the home with personal care (such as hygiene and exercise) and light household duties (such as meal preparation) and who monitors the patient's condition.[30]

IT, or *Information Technology*, when used in this field, should refer to *Healthcare Information Technology* (**HIT**, **HCIT**, or **HC-IT**) and includes anything related to computing technology, such as networking, hardware, software, the Internet, or the people who work with these technologies.

LPN. *Licensed Practical Nurse.*[31]

Medical Application. Computer software used in a health care organization; can include software that connects to medical devices such as hearing aids, medical imaging systems, remote patient monitoring and diagnostics, and medical alarm applications.

---

[29] Wikipedia web site. "Health Insurance Portability and Accountability Act."

[30] Dictionary.com web site. "Home health aide."

[31] Wikipedia web site. "Certified Nursing Assistant."

Medical Financial Applications Specialist. One who analyzes and defines financial management, project systems functions, business processes, and user needs; also analyzes and evaluates existing business functions and processes related to general accounting, accounts receivable/payable, inventory, budget, and procurement activities.[32]

Medical Records. Confidential documents that contain detailed and comprehensive information on an individual as well as the care and experience related to that person.

Medical Software System. Fully integrated system that allows access to scheduling, transcription, and document management for any health care office.

MPI. The *Master Patient Index*, utilized to track various **MRNs**.

MRN. A *Medical Record Number* is a patient's ID number at a medical institution.

NCVHS. *The National Committee on Vital and Health Statistics.*

NHIN. *The National Health Information Network.*

PANs. *Personal Account Numbers.*

Patient Care. Services rendered by members of the health profession, and nonprofessionals under their supervision, for the benefit of the patient.

PHI. *Protected Health Information.*

Project Management. Management of Information Technology projects. Planning and execution of any project from start to finish.

---

[32] Waller, 2010.

Proxy. An intermediary (that is, middle-man or go-between) for requests between a workstation and another server. The proxy acts as a filter for information, delivering only what was within the request description.

Requirements. Definitions for a given piece of software, based on functionality needed by its users.

RHIA. *Registered Health Information Administrator*, a position which usually requires a **CHIA** (Certificate in Health Information Administration).

Role. Description of what any system or program is designed to do.

Server. Computer system or application program that provides services to multiple computers and users.

Software. Programs and data held in the storage of a computer and used to direct the operation of the computer, as well as any documentation that provides instructions on how to use those programs.[33]

SSN. A person's *Social Security Number*.

Super User. On many computer operating systems, the super user, or root, is a special user account used for system administration.[34] This account has access to everything on the system and is not constrained by authorization levels.

TCO. The *total cost of ownership* of a given project, process, device, or institution.

---

[33] WordIQ web site. "Software Definition."
[34] Wikipedia web site. "Superuser."

Affiliates

The author wishes to thank the Health Care Information Technology Service Center (HC-IT-SC) and the Information Technology Center (ITC) for their affiliation with this project and for their generous support.

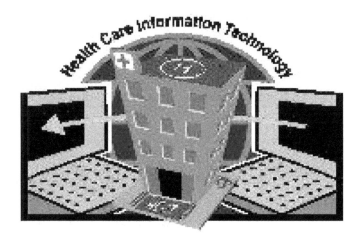

Feedback

The book you hold in your hands is part of a series intended to give professionals the most useful and up-to-date information necessary to ensure satisfactory outcomes in the field of Health Care IT. However, our ability to provide this information is greatly shaped by the invaluable feedback of our readers.

We welcome your suggestions, comments, and recommendations for future books in this series. Your input allows us to better serve your specific needs as we continue to publish additional information. We would be honored if you'd share with us what you'd like to see!

Please send all comments and suggestions to:

HC-IT-SC
Re: Book Feedback
P.O. Box 3388
Federal Way, WA 98063

References

1.   Summers W. Computer networks: Chapter 12—The network development life cycle. Columbus State University web site. Updated 17 July 2011. Accessed October 2010. http://csc.columbusstate.edu/summers/notes/cs457/chapt12.htm

2.   MerchantOS web site. The history of the computer. Updated 2010. Accessed 13 October 2010. http://www.merchantos.com/articles/informational/the-history-of-the-computer/

3.   Wikipedia web site. Health information management. Updated 28 July 2011. Accessed 13 October 2010. http://en.wikipedia.org/wiki/Health_information_management

4.   Wikipedia web site. Health information management. Updated 28 July 2011. Accessed 13 October 2010. http://en.wikipedia.org/wiki/Health_information_management

5.   Neal H. EHR vs. EMR–What's the difference? Software Advice web site. Updated 14 November 2008. Accessed 13 October 2010. http://www.softwareadvice.com/articles/medical/ehr-vs-emr-whats-the-difference/

6.   U.S. Department of Health and Human Services web site. Understanding health information privacy. Updated 2010. Accessed 12 June 2010. http://www.hhs.gov/ocr/privacy/hipaa/understanding/index.html

7.   US Innovation web site. The Obama-Biden plan. Updated 27 November 2008. Accessed 16 January 2011. http://www.usinnovation.org/files/ObamaTransitionTechAgenda112708.pdf

8.   Von Bergen, JM. Medical data breach said to be major. *The Philadelphia Inquirer*. Accessed 21 October 2010. http://www.philly.com/inquirer/business/20101021_Medical-data_breach_said_to_be_major.html

9.	Ponemon L. Annual study: Cost of a data breach. The Ponemon Institute web site. Updated January 2009. Accessed January 2010. http://www.ponemon.org/local/upload/fckjail/generalcontent/18/file/2008-2009%20US%20Cost%20of%20Data%20Breach%20Report%20Final.pdf

10.	Nicastro D. Data breaches cost hospitals $6B yearly. Health Leaders Media web site. Updated 5 November 2010. Accessed November 2010. http://www.healthleadersmedia.com/content/TEC-258666/Data-Breaches-Cost-Hospitals-6B-Yearly.html##

11.	Hennessy-Fiske M. Six California hospitals fined for medical record security breaches. *The Los Angeles Times*. Accessed 19 November 2010. http://articles.latimes.com/2010/nov/20/local/la-me-1120-hospital-fines-20101120

12.	Kahn JG. Billing and insurance-related administrative costs: Burden to health care providers. The University of California web site. Updated 21 May 2009. Accessed November 2010. http://www.iom.edu/~/media/Files/Activity%20Files/Quality/VSRT/Kahn 1.pdf

13.	Hartman T. Beacon Partners study reveals the progress healthcare organizations are making toward meaningful use. The Beacon Partners web site. Updated 19 November 2010. Accessed November 2010. http://www.beaconpartners.com/press_room/pressreleases/10/111810.htm

14.	Wikipedia web site. Certified nursing assistant. Updated 29 July 2011. Accessed 18 October 2010. http://en.wikipedia.org/wiki/Certified_nursing_assistant

15.	Wikipedia web site. Application analyst. Updated 29 November 2010. Accessed 18 October 2010. http://en.wikipedia.org/wiki/Application_analyst

16.	Business Dictionary web site. Business system. Updated 2010. Accessed 18 October 2010. http://www.businessdictionary.com/definition/business-system.html

17.	Thefreedictionary.com web site. Cellphone. Updated 2011. Accessed 18 October 2010. http://www.thefreedictionary.com/cellphone

18.	Muchira M. Cellphone technician job description. eHow web site. Updated 2011. Accessed 18 October 2010.

http://www.ehow.com/about_6722228_cell-phone-technician-job-description.html

19. Wikipedia web site. Certified nursing assistant. Updated 29 July 2011. Accessed 18 October 2010.
http://en.wikipedia.org/wiki/Certified_nursing_assistant

20. Thefreedictionary.com web site. CPT Codes. Updated 2011. Accessed 18 October 2010. http://medical-dictionary.thefreedictionary.com/CPT+codes

21. Thefreedictionary.com web site. CPT Codes. Updated 2011. Accessed 18 October 2010. http://medical-dictionary.thefreedictionary.com/CPT+codes

22. Neal H. EHR vs. EMR–What's the difference? Software Advice web site. Updated 14 November 2008. Accessed 13 October 2010. http://www.softwareadvice.com/articles/medical/ehr-vs-emr-whats-the-difference/

23. Neal H. EHR vs. EMR–What's the difference? Software Advice web site. Updated 14 November 2008. Accessed 13 October 2010. http://www.softwareadvice.com/articles/medical/ehr-vs-emr-whats-the-difference/

24. Open Projects web site. Computer hardware definition. Updated 2010. Accessed 18 October 2010. http://www.openprojects.org/hardware-definition.htm

25. Cahaba Government Benefits Administrators web site. Glossary of definitions: HCPCS code. Updated 24 May 2007. Accessed 18 October 2010. https://www.cahabagba.com/glossary/definitions/content1n9.htm

26. Ahima web site. Health information careers: Glossary of terms. Updated 2011. Accessed 18 October 2010. http://hicareers.com/Health_Information_101/glossary.aspx

27. U.S. Department of Health and Human Services web site. Understanding health information privacy. Updated 2010. Accessed 12 June 2010.

28. Wikipedia web site. Hearing Aid. Updated 19 July 2011. Accessed 18 October 2010. http://en.wikipedia.org/wiki/Hearing_aid

29. Wikipedia web site. Health Insurance Portability and Accountability Act. Updated 28 July 2011. Accessed 18 October 2010. http://en.wikipedia.org/wiki/Health_Insurance_Portability_and_Accountability_Act

30. Dictionary.com web site. Home health aide. Updated 2007. Accessed 18 October 2010. http://dictionary.reference.com/browse/home+health+aide

31. Wikipedia web site. Certified nursing assistant. Updated 29 July 2011. Accessed 18 October 2010. http://en.wikipedia.org/wiki/Certified_nursing_assistant

32. Waller R. Job description of an applications specialist. eHow web site. Updated 11 August 2010. Accessed 18 October 2010. http://www.ehow.com/about_6835027_job-description-application-specialist.html

33. WordIQ web site. Software definition. Updated 2010. Accessed 18 October 2010. http://www.wordiq.com/definition/Software

34. Wikipedia web site. Superuser. Updated 11 May 2011. Accessed 19 October 2010. http://en.wikipedia.org/wiki/Superuser

Further Reading

Business balls web site. Business process modeling. Updated 2009. Accessed 1[4] July 2010. http://www.businessballs.com/business-process-modelling.htm#BPMdefinition

Clements P, Bachmann F, Bass L, Garlan D, Ivers J, Little R, Nord R, and Stafford J. *Documenting software architectures–Views and beyond.* Boston, MA: Addison Wesley; 2003.

Healthposts.com.au web site. Health information manager. Updated 2005. Accessed 13 October 2010. http://www.healthposts.com.au/job/health-information-manager_1000.htm

HHS: National Committee on Vital and Health Statistics web site. Existing Medical Record Number (MRN) based identification. Updated 24 May 1999. Accessed 14 October 2010. http://www.ncvhs.hhs.gov/app7-8.htm

I2b2 web site. i2b2: Informatics for integrating biology and the bedside. Updated 1 June 2007. Accessed 4 August 2010. https://www.i2b2.org/resrcs/hive.html

Kruchten P. The '4+1' view model of software architecture. IBM web site. Updated November 1995. Accessed October 2010. http://www3.software.ibm.com/ibmdl/pub/software/rational/web/whitepapers/2003/Pbk4p1.pdf

Kulkarni A. Accounting terms–Glossary of accounting terms and definitions. Buzzle.com web site. Updated 2011. Accessed 12 June 2010. http://www.buzzle.com/articles/accounting-terms-glossary-of-accounting-terms-and-definitions.html

Object Management Group web site. UML 2.0 specification. Updated 2011. Accessed August 2010. http://www.omg.org/technology/documents/formal/uml.htm

PACS Admin web site. PACS administrators registry and certification association. Updated 2011. Accessed 12 June 2010. http://www.pacsadmin.org/

Pan J. Software testing. Carnegie Melon University web site. Updated 1999. Accessed 12 June 2010. http://www.ece.cmu.edu/~koopman/des_s99/sw_testing/#concepts

ProcessMaker.com web site. ProcessMaker is your open source BPM software solution. Updated 2010. Accessed 12 June 2010. http://www.processmaker.com/

Straube DM. HPCPS codes: Frequently asked questions. NLS.org web site. Updated November 2008. Accessed 12 June 2010 http://www.nls.org/av/FAQ%27s%20HCPCS.pdf

TM Floyd & Company web site. ICD-10 compliance: Building better solutions. Updated 2011. Accessed 18 October 2010. http://www.icd-10compliance.com/factors.asp

Tran E. Verification/Validation/Certification. Carnegie Melon University web site. Updated 1999. Accessed 14 June 2010. http://www.ece.cmu.edu/~koopman/des_s99/verification/

Wikipedia web site. Biba model. Updated 3 April 2011. Accessed 12 June 2010. http://en.wikipedia.org/wiki/Biba_model

Wikipedia web site. Health information technology. October 2010. Updated 22 April 2011. Accessed 13 October 2010.

http://en.wikipedia.org/wiki/Health_information_technology#Concepts_and_Definitions

Wikipedia web site. Micro instrumentation and telemetry systems. Updated 31 July 2011. Accessed 18 October 2010. http://en.wikipedia.org/wiki/Micro_Instrumentation_and_Telemetry_Systems.